Fitness Revolution

A Guide to Starting a Successful Gym or Personal Training Service

Table of Contents

Chapter 1. Introduction

Welcome to an exhilarating journey into the world of fitness entrepreneurship! "Fitness Revolution: A Guide to Starting a Successful Gym or Personal Training Service" is a comprehensive special report designed to ignite your passion, invigorate your business savvy and inspire you to create a thriving fitness venture. This resource is packed with essential tips and strategies meticulously curated from industry experts, successful gym owners, and reputed personal trainers. Whether you're just starting out on your fitness entrepreneur journey or you're a seasoned professional looking for innovative growth strategies, this inspiring guide will empower, engage, and encourage you towards constructing a profitable and sustainable fitness business. Get ready to pump up your business muscles and join the fitness revolution!

Chapter 2. Introduction to the Fitness Industry and Business Landscape

There has been a radical transformation in how society perceives fitness and wellness, given the mounting emphasis on health in our everyday lives. Our collective changing attitudes, driven by an increased understanding of the intricate relationship between lifestyle and overall well-being, has created a vibrant market landscape for fitness businesses.

2.1. A brief history of the Fitness Industry

In its early days, the fitness industry was predominantly composed of gymnasiums and health clubs, initially targeted at athletes and bodybuilders. However, as scientific discovery soared, it became clear that regular physical activity was a key component of maintaining optimum health for everyone. The industry has since diversified to include a myriad of different offerings, not limited to traditional gym circuits and loaded weights. It now encapsulates everything from cardio machines to yoga studios, personal training services to online fitness programs, dance classes to martial arts centers, and much more.

By the 1980s, the fitness industry had become a significant socio-economic trend in the West, soon spreading globally. It was during this period that it evolved into formal business structures. With growing consumer demand and a promising market, entrepreneurs quickly realized the potential for profitable ventures in this field.

2.2. Understanding the Modern Fitness Landscape

Now, the modern fitness industry exemplifies diversity with a range of businesses designed to cater to consumer preferences. As we transitioned into a new millennium, we saw a rise in niche gyms, 24/7 gym access, low-cost and luxury fitness clubs, and the emergence of boutique fitness studios, offering specialty classes to attract a specific clientele.

The fitness industry also saw a shift in its marketing approach. With the rise of social media, fitness marketing went digital, utilizing influencers to advertise health and fitness products, and offering online memberships, virtual classes, and personalized workout regimens.

Moreover, evolving technology has played a significant role in transforming the industry. The use of wearables, fitness apps, and equipment with integrated digital technology has empowered people to track their fitness progress, set achievable goals, and encourage steady motivation.

2.3. The Business Aspect of Fitness

As in any industry, successful fitness entrepreneurship is as much about the business acumen involved as it is about the services provided. Understanding the business environment; acclimating to its unique challenges, complexity, competition, and market conditions; and devising counter strategies accordingly are essential elements for success in the fitness sector.

To start a fitness business, you need a keen understanding of your target demographic – HR managers considering corporate wellness programs, beginner-level yoga attendees, or fitness-savvy millennials looking for premium training experiences, for instance. Additionally, your marketing and sales strategy, pricing model, and your unique value proposition must reflect these demographic preferences.

Operational efficiency is paramount. This means competent workforce management, budgeting, timely service delivery, top-notch equipment maintenance, and ensuring an inspiring environment for your clientele to continue their fitness journey.

2.4. Trending Opportunities in the Fitness Industry

The fitness landscape presents abundant entrepreneurial opportunities. With the advent of the COVID-19 pandemic, the industry saw a precipitous rise in at-home workouts indicating a promising future for virtual personal trainers and fitness apps.

Another increasing trend is the focus on holistic wellness, where businesses offer not just exercise routines but also nutritional advice, mental health support, and lifestyle management. Inclusivity-focused fitness spaces, designed to cater to different ages, abilities, and fitness levels, are also on the rise.

Meanwhile, corporate wellness programs present another prosperous avenue as more companies recognize the benefits of investing in employee health and productivity.

2.5. Final Word

We are witnessing an exciting era in the fitness industry filled with a wide array of opportunities coupled with emerging challenges. Sophisticated customer expectations, intense market competition, and the continuously evolving sector demand that budding entrepreneurs not just be fitness fanatics, but also astute business strategists.

Embrace this journey with an open mind, eagerness to learn, and tolerance for trial-and-error. As you dive deeper into subsequent sections of this guide, you'll discover invaluable insights into establishing a lucrative fitness business that resonates with your target audience, stands against competition, and influences positive change in the lives of many.

Your venture into fitness entrepreneurship is not just a business initiative; it's a commitment to enhancing societal wellness. And that in itself is a victory worth striving for. So let's move forward, dive deeper, and embrace the fitness revolution!

Chapter 3. Assessing Your Vision: Crafting Your Unique Fitness Proposition

Before diving headfirst into your fitness entrepreneurship journey, it is crucial to start from within. Understanding your vision, your purpose, and your unique offering will lay the foundation for a sustainable and successful fitness business. This chapter will guide you through that process, beginning with the articulation of your vision.

3.1. Understanding Your Vision

Your vision comprises the core purpose of your business and an ideal depiction of what you aspire for it to become. It's a peek into the future, a dream you have for your enterprise's development and growth. But why is a vision important? Aside from serving as a guiding light to your business decisions, it inspires motivation, enhances team cooperation, and helps in establishing your business's unique identity.

To formulate your vision, reflect on what your ideal fitness business looks like. What kind of culture does it breed? What values does it embody? What unique experience does it provide to its clients? Write down as much as you can, no matter how far-fetched or challenging they may seem.

3.2. Crafting Your Unique Fitness Proposition

Identifying your Unique Fitness Proposition (UFP) is a pivotal step in setting your business apart. It's what makes your gym or personal training service distinct from numerous other fitness businesses.

To start crafting your UFP, consider your target demographic. Who do you aspire to help? Novice gym-goers? Elite athletes, elderly individuals, or youth? Or perhaps your focus is broader, encompassing everyone interested in a healthier lifestyle?

Next, ask yourself what specific service or benefit you can offer. Are you providing personalized training, group classes, or a distinct method of training? Are you offering services for rehabilitation, weight loss, strength building, or holistic well-being?

Finally, decide how you can serve your clients better than anyone else. Do you have exclusive equipment, a conducive environment, experienced staff, an effective training program? Your UFP should respond to customer needs and differentiate you from the competition.

3.3. Merging Your Vision and UFP

With a vision and UFP in hand, it's time to blend both elements. Having a clear vision centered around your UFP increases your chances of creating an impactful and successful fitness business.

Identify how your UFP can be enhanced or supported by your vision. What aspects of your vision are directly tied to your UFP? The synergy between your vision and UFP should be seamless, each supporting and strengthening the other.

3.4. Vision-Driven Branding

Branding is not just about your business name and logo; it involves your overall business image and how it appeals to your target audience. A strong, vision-driven brand captivates, motivates, and ultimately persuades people to choose your fitness business over your competitors.

To formulate a vision-driven brand, consider how your business vision reflects in your name, logo, slogan, and even your interior design. Your company's every aspect should convey your vision and UFP.

3.5. Creating Your Fitness Entrepreneur Story

A compelling story gives your fitness business an emotional impact. It personifies your business and makes it relatable. Your story might be about your personal fitness journey, the reason behind why you started your fitness business, or the difference you plan to make in people's lives.

Weave your story around your vision and UFP. Let it communicate the passion behind your vision and the benefit of your UFP to clients. Embed this story in every aspect of your business, from your website to your social media presence and customer interactions.

3.6. Assessing Your Vision: A Checklist

We conclude this chapter with a checklist that will help you assess your vision and refine your UFP:

1. Does your vision paint a vivid picture of your desired future?

2. Is your UFP distinct, addressing a specific niche or offering a unique service?

3. Does a seamless synergy exist between your vision and UFP, mutually enhancing both?

4. Does your branding visually and emotionally reflect your vision and UFP?

5. Does your story evoke emotions, embody your vision, and reinforce your UFP?

The time you spend assessing your vision and crafting your UFP will pay dividends as you lay the groundwork for your distinctive fitness business. This foundational work will not only affect all of your business decisions but also will help create a compelling identity that resonates with and attracts your desired client base.

This chapter is your first step in the exciting journey of becoming an innovative fitness business owner, the first pump of the iron as you strengthen and tone the muscles of your budding business. Be bold, cultivate resilience, and harness your entrepreneurial spirit as you rise in fitness revolution.

Chapter 4. Location Magic: Selecting and Securing the Perfect Spot

The first critical step on your entrepreneurial journey in the fitness industry is finding the perfect location for your gym or personal training service. The significance of this phase cannot be overstressed - your chosen spot significantly influences your business's visibility, accessibility, and overall success.

4.1. Research Your Market

The initial step in pinpointing the perfect spot for your fitness business is to conduct extensive market research. Understand the demographics and fitness habits of your target customers. Familiarize yourself with your competitors and their locations. Are there certain areas where fitness facilities are clustered? If so, consider whether there is room for another gym or whether it might be advantageous to set up shop in an underserved neighborhood.

Gain insights from population density statistics. Affluent, densely populated areas often spell lucrative opportunities for gyms and fitness services.

4.2. Evaluate Accessibility and Visibility

Location visibility and accessibility significantly influence your gym's foot traffic. A gym located in a bustling, high-visibility location invariably secures more memberships than a gym obscured in a difficult-to-reach alley.

Choose a location that's easy for your potential clients to find and reach. Good examples might include commercial areas, shopping centers, or popular commuting routes with ample parking or public transport links.

4.3. Consider Space Needs

When estimating space needs for your fitness business, consider the types of services you will be offering. Your space requirements will be vastly different if you plan to operate a compact, high-intensity interval training (HIIT) gym as opposed to a sprawling fitness center with an Olympic-sized pool.

Similarly, personal training studios do not demand as much space as traditional gyms but require a more personalized and comfortable setting.

Consider future expansion possibilities too. Starting from a small location is perfectly fine, as long as you keep an eye open for scalable places.

4.4. Analyze Costs

Be cautious in balancing the trade-off between location effectiveness and rental costs. While a high-traffic and upscale location can potentially attract more clients initially, it will also likely bear a premium price. Conduct a thorough cost-benefit analysis before making a decision.

Cost considerations should extend beyond mere rental charges. Additional expenses could include property taxes, insurance, utilities, and parking facilities. Be sure these costs can be supported comfortably within your budget before deciding on a place.

4.5. Inspect Infrastructure Quality

Before signing a lease or purchasing a property, thoroughly inspect the condition of the building.

Visit the site multiple times at different hours to understand its natural lighting, noise backgrounds, and overall ambiance. Consider facilities like showers, restrooms, and changing rooms.

If you're buying a previously-used gym, assess the state of the current equipment and whether refurbishment or replacement is necessary.

4.6. Legal and Zoning Conditions

Before settling on a spot, ensure you understand the pertinent building codes, zoning laws, and any restrictions that might affect a gym's operation. Sometimes, residential neighborhoods may have regulations that restrict the operation of businesses.

You'll also want to verify whether you need specific permits or licenses to operate a gym in your selected location. All these legal considerations, though tedious, can shield you from future legal complications or unexpected fines.

4.7. Lease Agreement Nuances

Once you've zeroed in on the perfect spot for your fitness venture, you will have to tackle real estate lease agreements. This could be a straightforward process or a convoluted one, depending on the terms and conditions.

Negotiate terms that favor you - whether it's regarding lease duration, rent amount, or specifics about property enhancements. Engaging a professional negotiator or legal counsel can prove beneficial during this process.

To conclude, securing the perfect spot for your fitness business is a blend of strategic planning, thorough analysis, and patience. Your chosen space will play a pivotal role in influencing the appeal and profitability of your venture. Make this decision with care, as the right location is indeed magic for your fitness business.

Chapter 5. Crunching the Numbers: Initial Investment, Maintenance, and Projections

It's often said that numbers don't lie. In the domain of fitness entrepreneurship, this adage holds more relevance than ever. A clear grasp of your financial landscape—the initial investment required, ongoing maintenance costs, and future financial projections—is not just crucial but foundational to your venture's success.

5.1. Initial Investment

The proverbial first step into the world of fitness entrepreneurship begins with the analysis of the initial investment. This investment can be divided into several primary categories: infrastructure and equipment, staff salaries, marketing, technology, and licensing or permits.

1. Infrastructure and Equipment

The base of any gym or personal training service is its infrastructure. This includes the physical location—either leasing or buying a property, renovations, and the purchase of gym equipment. According to the International Health, Racquet, & Sportsclub Association (IHRSA), the gym equipment alone for a boutique fitness studio can cost between $10,000 to $50,000. For larger, comprehensive fitness centers, this cost can run upwards from $100,000.

1. Staff Salaries

Trained and professional personnel are the backbone of your gym or personal training service. This category includes personal trainers, nutritionists, gym managers, administrative and cleaning staff. Their salaries and associated costs often represent a significant portion of the initial outlay.

1. Marketing

No business can thrive without effective marketing. This includes online advertising, print media, and outdoor advertisements, all aimed at attracting your target clientele. This also encapsulates costs related to website development and maintenance, social media management, and local outreach initiatives.

1. Technology

Modern gyms thrive on technology. On the one hand, one needs fitness equipment like treadmills and stationary bikes with digital interfaces. Additionally, gym management software for scheduling, billing, and CRM (Customer Relationship Management) cannot be overlooked.

1. Licensing and Permits

Fitness centers require specific licenses and permits, which also require a budget. This includes health department permits, sign permits, resale permits, building permits, and potentially more depending on your location.

5.2. Maintenance Costs

Once your door is open, your attention must shift to ongoing maintenance costs. Ignoring these routine expenses can result in unforeseen financial turmoil.

1. Equipment Upgrades and Maintenance

Fitness equipment is not a one-time investment. Even with regular servicing, these equipment pieces need replacement every 5 to 7 years on average. Moreover, potential repairs and routine maintenance must be considered in the budget.

1. Utility Bills

Water, electricity, heating, and air conditioning are ongoing utilities expenses that can't be overlooked. Remember, a gym often consumes more electricity than a typical office or commercial space due to continuous running of fitness equipment, and often extended operating hours.

1. Rent and Salary Increases

Both rent and salaries usually increase over time. Allocating a percentage increase per year in your financial planning can save from nasty surprises down the line.

1. Marketing

Similar to the initial investment phase, marketing remains an ongoing cost. Advertising, website maintenance and updates, SEO, social media campaigns, promotional offers, and customer retention efforts – they all continue to require a steady cash flow.

1. Miscellaneous Expenses

This includes any unexpected costs, like emergency repairs, changes in licensing regulations, legal fees, and more.

5.3. Projections

Given the varying nature of the fitness sector, making financial projections is not an exact science. However, a conservative approach would be to consider all of the above costs, a reasonable time-frame for profitability, and studying comparable models in the market.

Estimating revenue requires a careful evaluation of member acquisition costs, expected member retention rate, pricing strategy, and additional income streams such as merchandise sales, on-site nutrition bar sales, or personal training packages.

Though challenging, establishing a successful fitness business venture remains achievable with a robust financial plan in place. As you're crunching the numbers, remember to plan for the unpredictable and keep space for adjustment and adaptability. The road to fitness entrepreneurship may be a steep climb, but with a firm grip on your financial landscape, the view from the top is indeed worth it.

Whether you're going to establish the next trendy fitness boutique or a comprehensive, full-service fitness center, use these monetary calculations as your roadmap for success, not a deterrent. With this solid financial blueprint in hand, you're that much closer to joining the ranks of successful fitness entrepreneurs. Let the fitness revolution begin!

Chapter 6. Fit Out Your Fitness Centre: Choosing the Right Equipment

It's often said that the equipment you choose for your gym is the heart and soul of your facility. Selecting the most suitable setup can directly impact your fitness centre's success. It's no easy task and involves comprehensive consideration of your budget, target market, space constraints, and fitness training style.

6.1. Assessing Your Needs

Firstly, determine your objective and the demographic you intend to serve. A thorough understanding of your clientele's workout needs, fitness goals, and preferences will aid in procuring the right equipment. Are your members predominantly young gym-goers looking for weight training? Or are they seniors focusing on balance and flexibility? Perhaps your clientele favours group training, or maybe they're primarily inclined towards high-intensity interval training (HIIT)? These factors significantly influence your equipment choices. If your gym specialises in cardio workouts, ensure that you invest heavily in treadmills, ellipticals, stationary bikes, and rowers. Alternatively, strength training equipment such as barbells, dumbbells, weight plates, and resistance machines should dominate your space if you're focusing on weightlifting or bodybuilding workouts.

6.2. Budget Consideration

A careful evaluation of your financial status will give you a clear picture of the funds available to buy equipment. Remember, more expensive doesn't necessarily mean better. Make sure to get high-quality pieces that can withstand heavy usage and are low on maintenance instead of opting for ones with fancy add-ons that might seldom be used. Consider both new and secondhand equipment. Pre-owned equipment can be an economical choice, especially for bootstrapping start-ups. If cost remains a constraint, leasing options can be explored.

6.3. Spatial Planning

Planning your fitness centre's layout for optimal workflow and safety will guide you on the kind and amount of equipment that can be accommodated. A well-designed gym layout optimises space, accommodates a variety of workout zones, facilitates easy navigation, and supports efficient equipment cleaning and maintenance. Here you can follow the 60-40 rule, which suggests that 60% of your space should be allocated for cardio and weight training equipment, and 40% should be left as an open space for functional training, group classes, and free weights.

6.4. Selecting Your Equipment

The types of equipment you choose will depend on the training programs you plan to offer. A basic starting list might include:

- Cardio machines like treadmills, ellipticals, stationary bikes

- Strength equipment such as resistance machines, dumbbells, barbells, kettlebells, and weight plates

- Functional/Flexibility tools like yoga mats, resistance bands, medicine balls, and foam rollers

- Speciality equipment for specific training such as rowing machines, punching bags, TRX bands depending on your gym's focus

While purchasing, considerations must be given to the durability, warranty, and maintenance requirements of each piece.

6.5. Vendor Selection

Choosing a trusted and reliable vendor plays a crucial role in the selection of the right equipment. Look for industry-reputed brands known for their quality. Read reviews, examine their after-sales service, and enquire about any possible additional services such as installation, maintenance, and repair. Always ensure to buy CE-marked equipment that complies with standards and regulations for safety.

6.6. Implementing Technology

In the modern fitness world, integrating technology has become increasingly significant. Technologically advanced equipment like smart treadmills and stationary bikes can offer users a better workout experience and give your gym a competitive edge.

6.7. Regular Maintenance and Upgrades

Regular upkeep of gym equipment extends their lifespan and guarantees the safety of users. Establish a maintenance schedule to keep your equipment in top condition. Keeping up with industry trends and continuously upgrading your equipment is essential to ensure your facility stays up-to-date.

Choosing the right equipment is a fundamental step in the creation of a successful fitness centre. Balancing cost, space, user needs, and safety will enable you to curate a fitness environment that not only meets the workout necessities of your members but also provides an ethos and atmosphere conducive to well-being and fitness progress.

Chapter 7. Building a Kickass Team: Hiring and Training Staff

Building an effective team for your fitness enterprise is integral to the success and growth of your business. Not only does a powerful team help deliver exceptional service, but it also aids in influencing customer loyalty and retention.

7.1. Understanding Your Team's Role

Before you begin the hiring process, it's essential to understand the roles your team will need to fulfill. These responsibilities could range from personal trainers and group class instructors to receptionists and maintenance staff depending on the scale and structure of your fitness venture. Each member of your team will be crucial to your daily operations, contributing to the overall client experience.

7.2. Hiring the Right People

Hiring the right set of individuals for your team is the next step. Begin by creating detailed job descriptions for each position, outlining skills, qualifications, and experience you're looking for. Be sure to highlight the values and ethos of your fitness brand to attract candidates who share your vision.

Your team should comprise expert professionals who share your passion for health and fitness. Scan through the applicant's certifications and endorsements from recognized fitness bodies such as the National Strength and Conditioning Association (NSCA) or

American Council on Exercise (ACE).

Try to look beyond their technical expertise and evaluate their interpersonal and customer service skills – essential traits for maintaining a loyal clientele in the fitness industry. Coaching is about developing a relationship, and you'll need individuals who can adapt to varying client personalities while ensuring they remain encouraged and motivated towards their fitness goals.

7.3. Training Your Team

Once you've hired the right individuals, the next step is to focus on their training and development. Every gym and fitness center operates differently. Even experienced staff might need guidance to adapt to your specific ways of handling operations, client management, and even crisis situations. Training is the opportune time to communicate your brand's philosophy, operational protocol, and service standards, establishing a unified entity that moves and evolves together.

Regular in-house workshops and seminars are a fabulous investment. Bring in specialists or established names in the industry to refresh your staff's knowledge and keep them updated with the latest trends and techniques.

7.4. Maintaining Staff Morale

Staff morale plays a crucial role in the overall customer experience. A motivated and enthusiastic team will channel their positive energy to their clients, fostering a vibrant and energetic environment, translating into client retention and referrals.

Periodic appreciation in the form of awards and recognitions, a fair system of incentives and bonuses, open and clear communication, and scope for task autonomy can foster a sense of satisfaction among your staff, leading to increased productivity and commitment.

7.5. Investing in Your Team

Remember, your team is not just a cost to your business; they're an investment. You might have the most advanced equipment and facilities, but without a proficient and enthusiastic team, your venture may struggle. Invest in your team's growth and development just as you would your personal. Encouraging your team to acquire higher qualifications, certifying in new fitness disciplines, or specialize in niche workout techniques are ways to bringing enhanced value to your services.

In conclusion, building a kickass team is not just about hiring; it's a meticulous process involving understanding your needs, selecting the right professionals, training them according to your brand vision, maintaining a motivated work culture, and continuously investing in their growth and learning.

Remember, your team reflects your brand. By investing in their capacities, confidence, and care, you go a long way towards ensuring the success and durability of your fitness venture. It's a continuous cycle of learning, evolving, and growing together - that's how you build a team that makes your fitness business kickass.

Chapter 8. Creating the Buzz: Marketing Strategies That Work

Venturing into a fitness business can be a thrilling endeavor, fraught with possibilities and potential. However, to truly stand out in a saturated market and attract a steady influx of clients, you need to 'create the buzz' through powerful marketing strategies. This section provides a detailed roadmap to navigate the complex and ever-changing landscape of fitness marketing.

8.1. Understanding Your Niche

Before devising any marketing tactics, you need to comprehend your niche. Knowing your target audience, their interests, needs, and behaviors will contribute to more efficient and impactful marketing strategies.

Define your preferred clientele, are they fitness beginners, seasoned bodybuilders, or perhaps interested in yoga or Pilates? Are they looking for personal training or group classes? Understanding the demographic and psychographic characteristics of your market will form the foundation of all your marketing decisions.

8.2. Designing a Compelling Brand

Your brand is far more than just your logo or tagline. It's an amalgamation of your vision, values, and unique selling proposition (USP) that shapes customer perceptions. Make your brand extraordinary, relatable, and unique.

Ask yourself, what makes your gym or personal training service different? Why should customers choose you over the competition? Be sure to embed your USP into every aspect of your branding and overtly communicate this to your audience.

8.3. Building a Strong Online Presence

In this digital era, having a noticeable online presence is paramount. A professional, user-friendly website with clear information about your services, pricing, and contact details is crucial. Enhancing your site's visibility with Search Engine Optimization (SEO) techniques and continuous content generation will also drive traffic to your site.

Social media platforms like Facebook, Instagram, Twitter, and LinkedIn are other great avenues to interact with your audience and build relationships. Regular updates, engaging posts, workout tips, client testimonials and success stories will keep your followers engaged and provide social proof.

8.4. Leveraging Email Marketing

Despite the domination of social media, email marketing still proves as a significant marketing platform with a high return on investment (ROI). Delivering personalized offers, helpful tips, and noteworthy news directly into the inboxes of your existing and prospective clients, you can build loyalty, increase retention, and provoke referrals.

Consider using an email marketing software like Mailchimp or Constant Contact to automate your messaging, and don't forget to include an enticing call-to-action in every mail.

8.5. Offering Free Trials or Introductory Offers

Free trials or discounted introductory offers are a common, yet effective strategy in the fitness world. Not only do they attract newbies but also provide an opportunity for them to assess your services and facilities. It's a win-win situation, as satisfied clients are likely to convert into full-time members.

8.6. Implementing a Referral Program

A referral program encourages your existing members to bring their friends, coworkers, or family members to your service, often in exchange for free workouts, discounts, or other perks. As clients tend to trust recommendations from people they know, this can be a powerful marketing tool.

8.7. Hosting Community Events

Hosting fitness challenges, open days, workshops, or partnering with local health fairs or charity runs can notably raise your brand awareness and introduce potential clients to your offering. These opportunities also allow your facility to build rapport within the local community as a supporter of healthy lifestyles.

8.8. Exploring Collaborations and Partnerships

Align with businesses that complement your services. Collaborations with healthy food restaurants, sports equipment stores, or physiotherapy clinics can open new channels to reach a wider audience and can lead to a mutually beneficial partnership.

8.9. Continual Learning and Adjusting

Remember, effective marketing requires consistent testing and adjusting. Track all your marketing initiatives, identify what works and what doesn't, and reiterate your strategies accordingly. This continual learning process will ensure your marketing efforts remain effective and fruitful throughout your business growth.

With these strategies on your marketing plan, you're well on your way to creating the buzz you need for your successful venture into fitness entrepreneurship. But remember, without exceptional service to back up your marketing, even the best strategies may fall flat. "Fitness Revolution: A Guide to Starting a Successful Gym or Personal Training Service" serves as a comprehensive tool to not just amplify your marketing prowess but also to hone your operational and customer service skills, laying a solid foundation for your robust fitness empire.

Chapter 9. Customer Service 101: Retaining and Expanding Clientele

Customer service in the fitness industry isn't simply about providing a pleasant experience for your members. It's about creating an unwavering bond between them and your fitness facility - a connection that ensures they consistently choose your services over the competition. From member retention to organic promotion through positive word-of-mouth, excellent customer service can enhance multiple aspects of your business.

9.1. The Pursuit of Excellence

Excellence in customer service should be the backbone of your fitness business. Achieving this goal requires a sense of decency, positivity, and professionalism. Remember that each client is unique, which means there isn't a one-size-fits-all solution. Building a client-centered model and tailoring your service to individual needs is the key to satisfaction.

To ensure excellence in customer service, you must have clear communication, empathy, and an understanding of your client's fitness goals. Regular check-ins and follow-ups reassure your clients that their progress and satisfaction are your top priorities. Moreover, it's essential to keep an open line for client feedback and criticism, allowing you to continually refine your services.

9.2. Building Strong Relationships

Developing strong relationships is crucial for client retention. One of the most effective ways to establish these bonds is through personalisation. Simple gestures like addressing clients by their first names or showing genuine interest in their fitness goals can make a big difference.

When it comes to managing relationships, emotional intelligence matters. Always remember each client's unique motivations, goals, progress, and challenges. Equipping your team of trainers and staff with the right communication skills will allow them to connect with clients on a deeper level.

Regularly survey your clientele to gain insights into their preferences and satisfaction level. This practice will highlight areas where your services are excelling and where there's room for improvement.

9.3. Retaining Existing Clients

It is generally more cost-effective to retain existing customers than to acquire new ones. As such, your focus on member retention should never waver.

Creating a friendly atmosphere is key to keeping clients hooked onto your gym or personal training service. The idea is to make clients feel like they're part of a community where they can comfortably work towards their fitness objectives.

In addition to general atmosphere, consider incentivizing longstanding membership through loyalty reward programs. Clients love being recognized for their loyalty, and something as simple as a discounted membership for loyal members can foster client retention.

9.4. Expanding Your Clientele

Increasing your client base is as important as retaining existing ones. To achieve this, leverage satisfied customers for referrals. Encourage them to spread the word about your stellar customer service. You can even offer rewards for each successful referral, creating a win-win situation for both parties.

Online platforms can also help in expanding your client base. Encourage happy customers to leave positive reviews on popular platforms like Google and Yelp. People often consider online reviews before selecting a gym or personal training service, and positive experiences can help you attract more clients.

9.5. Handling Complaints Positively

Complaints are unavoidable, but how you handle them can make or break your relationship with clients. Always acknowledge your client's concern and show empathy. It's better to apologize and rectify the situation than to argue or dismiss their feedback. In the end, the solution you come up with should leave your clients feeling heard and valued.

Remember, complaints can be constructive. They enable you to understand faults in your customer service and workout offerings that you might have overlooked, and address them promptly.

9.6. Staying Ahead with Innovation

Staying ahead in the fitness industry involves constant innovation. Monitor industry trends regularly to ensure your services remain up to date. Introduce new workouts, training techniques, or equipment periodically based on clients' fitness objectives and interests.

Offering digital solutions, like online booking and remote personal training services, can also enhance customer satisfaction. Not only do such services offer convenience, but they also cater to members who prefer at-home workouts.

9.7. Teaming Up for Success

Your team is an essential component of your customer service engine. Make sure they are well-versed with your customer service philosophy and values. Regular training on communication, empathy, and relationship-building can help your trainers and support staff deliver an unmatched customer experience.

To conclude, excellent customer service spans across several aspects of your business: achieving excellence, developing strong relationships, retaining clients, expanding clientele, handling complaints positively, staying innovative, and continual staff training. By focusing on these key areas, you can build a successful fitness business that continues to flourish.

Chapter 10. Risk Management: Insurance, Health Standards and Legal Compliance

Starting a fitness venture involves navigating numerous risks. These range from injuries that could occur on the premises, to compliance with health standards and legal requirements. As an entrepreneur, it's important that you thoroughly understand and manage these risks effectively to ensure the business can thrive and be sustainable long-term.

10.1. Understanding Your Risk Profile

It's crucial to first understand the different types of risks associated with running a fitness business – the potential for personal injury stands out. In the sport and fitness industry, the risk of bodily harm, whether minor or significant, is always present. This is due to the very physical nature of industry activities. Even with the utmost care and professionalism, accidents and injuries can happen.

Moreover, running a fitness space entails other risk factors, such as equipment failure, property damage, workplace-related illnesses, and even cyber threats if you handle customers' personal and payment information.

Once you identify the risks inherent in your business type, you can develop a systematic approach towards mitigating them, including prevention plans, risk-handling systems and effective insurance coverage.

10.2. Insurance: Types and Necessities

Insurance is a key component in risk management within the fitness industry. It provides a financial safety net against unforeseen events which could otherwise be crippling for the business. Let's explore the main types of insurance you should consider:

1. General Liability Insurance: This covers your business from a variety of claims, including injury, accidents, or claims of negligence. It can help pay for property damage, medical expenses, libel, slander, legal costs, and faulty products. Every fitness business should have this as a basic level of protection.

2. Professional Indemnity Insurance: This protects you if clients claim that your services have caused them harm, such as poor training advice or inappropriate exercise plan that led to injury.

3. Workers' Compensation Insurance: If you have employees, this insurance provides wage replacement and medical benefits to those who are injured while working. In exchange for these benefits, the employee gives up the rights to sue the business for negligence.

4. Equipment Insurance: As you know, fitness equipment can be expensive. This type of insurance covers damage or theft of your gym equipment.

5. Cyber Insurance: If you store sensitive client information, like credit card numbers, or work with online payment technologies, your business might be a target of cyber threats. Cyber insurance supports you in case of data breaches or other cyber incidents.

10.3. Health and Safety Standards

To mitigate personal injury risks, a comprehensive understanding of health and safety standards is absolutely essential. Health and safety procedures are foundational to the operation of a successful fitness business. These range from cleanliness and hygiene, equipment safety protocols, to first aid availability.

Often, governments provide detailed health and safety regulation for fitness facilities, which should be one of the first resources to consult when planning for this aspect. Next, take advantage of industry associations and their resources, many of which offer health and safety training programs, resources, and checklists to help fitness businesses maintain government and industry standards.

10.4. Managing Legal Compliance

In addition to health and safety regulations, fitness businesses also need to comply with various state, local and federal laws. Some of them include:

Zoning Laws: These laws regulate where businesses can operate. Make sure your establishment complies with local zoning ordinances before you sign a lease or purchase a property.

Employment Laws: If you plan to hire employees, you need to comply with various employment-related laws, such as wage requirements, discrimination laws, and workers' compensation rules.

Privacy Laws: As a fitness business, you'll be collecting, storing, and using personal information. Make sure your business complies with existing data protection and privacy laws.

Business Licensing: Different cities, states, or countries may require fitness centres to have specific business licenses. Check the local requirements and ensure your business has the necessary licenses and permits.

Contract Law: Fitness businesses usually facilitate their services through client agreements or membership contracts. Therefore, understanding contract law to create fair and legally sound contracts is critical.

In essence, to successfully navigate the world of fitness entrepreneurship, entrepreneur's foremost duties are understanding the inherent risks their business might face, adhering to the appropriate insurances, promoting a culture of health and safety, and maintaining legal compliance. Putting in the effort to manage these risks not only secures the business operation but also paves the way for a flourishing fitness venture.

Chapter 11. Growing Pains and Gains: Scaling Your Fitness Business for Success

Whether you're managing a flourishing gym or personal training service, focusing solely on maintaining the status quo can limit your business's potential. You've established a solid base, garnered a loyal client base, and now it's time to consider entering the next stage—scaling. Scaling involves expanding your operations efficiently to accommodate more clients, generate increased revenue, and boost profitability, all while maintaining exploratory high-quality services.

11.1. The Uphill Climb: Beginnings of Business Scaling

A common dilemma faced by successful fitness professionals is deciding when to scale their business. There's no one-size-fits-all answer because various elements such as market dynamics, existing resources, and individual goals play key roles in determining the right time.

Typically, a good indicator that you're ready to scale is when demand consistently outstrips your service's current capacity. Other signs could include consistent profits, steady cash flow, robust processes, and a stable, reliable team.

Scaling is not an overnight feat; it's an uphill climb. However, remember that every step, small or significant, moves you closer to your entrepreneurial summit.

11.2. Embracing Change: Transforming Business Operations

The first step towards scaling is, paradoxically, changing your mindset. Recognize and embrace that you'll need to transform aspects of your current operations. This could include investing in new fitness equipment, hiring additional team members, offering novel services, or even opening a new facility.

Next, examine your business model. Your current model has brought you success; however, that doesn't imply it will be successful in a larger operation. Changes may be necessary to generate consistent returns at the new scale. For example, consider group programming, virtual training, or corporate partnership packages if you haven't incorporated them yet.

11.3. Strategic Success: Business Expansion Planning

Strategic planning is a vital element to successful scaling. You'll need a detailed business plan that outlines your growth goals and the steps necessary to achieve them. This should include a market analysis, marketing and sales strategies, financial projections, and an action plan with timelines.

Your action plan is your roadmap to success, acting as a step-by-step guide to reaching your growth goals. This should include tasks like hiring and training staff, marketing strategies, budgeting, and facility expansions.

11.4. Investing in Human Capital: Team Building and Development

Scaling means dealing with more clients and potentially expanding your services. To meet this increased demand, you'll need a bigger, well-trained team.

Start by identifying the roles you need. Besides fitness trainers, roles such as customer service representatives, operations managers, cleaning staff, and marketing specialists may be imperative to executing an effective scaling strategy. Keep in mind that the right team can either make or break your scaling plan.

Continual employee development is also of paramount importance. Prioritize onboarding and training to ensure your team delivers excellent service, consistently. Recognize that expertise in fitness alone may not suffice—soft skills like communication, teamwork, and customer service are equally significant.

11.5. The Financial Aspect: Smart Budgeting and Funding

A key aspect of scaling is budgeting. It's essential to produce a detailed budget that precisely outlines your projected income and expenses.

Consider the costs for staff wages, equipment investment, renovation or relocation expenses, marketing campaigns, additional operational costs, and an emergency fund for unforeseen expenditures. Without this, any unplanned costs could spell disaster for your scaling plans.

Additionally, consider your funding options. Savings, business profits, personal loans, small business loans, angel investors, or even crowdfunding campaigns could be potential sources of capital.

11.6. Customer is King: Maintaining Service Excellence

As your fitness business grows, it's essential to retain your service quality. This involves continually monitoring and refining your services as necessary.

Consider ways to maintain engagement and rapport with each customer while simultaneously handling a larger clientele base. This could involve hiring a dedicated customer service team or implementing a reliable CRM system to manage customer relations effectively.

11.7. Metrics that Matter: Establishing Key Performance Indicators

Establishing Key Performance Indicators (KPIs) can help you monitor your business's performance and properly gauge your scaling success.

KPIs can consist of financial metrics, such as profit margins and revenue growth, or operational metrics, such as customer retention rates, customer satisfaction scores, or employee churn rates.

11.8. Measuring Success: Regular Audits and Feedback

Regularly evaluate your progress towards your scaling goals. This involves conducting periodical performance audits and seeking feedback from customers and team members.

Customer feedback is valuable for highlighting areas for improvement and evaluating if your service quality is consistent. Similarly, team feedback can provide insights into operational difficulties and potential areas of development.

Finally, don't forget that scaling is a journey. Appreciate the process, continually learn, adapt your strategy as required, and always strive for improvement. Remember that growth is a sign of life—embrace the pain that accompanies it as a token of progress and the inevitable gateway to future gain.